Mic

Gluten Free Desserts Recipes

51 Quick And Easy Recipes For Gluten-Free Desserts For The Whole Family

© Copyright 2021 by **Michelle Parker**

The photos of the recipes are indicative.

WARNING

The information in this book is for informational purposes only. It is not medical advice or medical opinion and should not be construed as such in any way. Before starting the Sirt diet or taking the foods and/or supplements recommended for this diet, always seek advice from a trusted physician or qualified nutritionist. This is essential to avoid possible side effects. We disclaim any responsibility for any ailments or problems should you decide to follow the Sirt diet or take any foods or supplements associated with this diet.

Table of Contents

Michelle Parker

Gluten Intolerance

Definition

Gluten intolerance is a Para physiological condition of altered intestinal tolerance to a protein nutrient, called gluten.

The term "celiac disease" or "c(o)eliac" comes from the greek "koiliakos κοιλιακός", which means "abdominal"; this term was introduced in 1800 to translate an ancient Greek description of the so-called disease of "Areteo of Cappadocia".

Gluten intolerance is NOT an allergy, neither to gluten, nor to other wheat proteins or the like.

While it is true that it involves the intervention of the immune system (like allergies), it is also true that celiac disease does so in a totally different way than allergic forms. Gluten intolerance causes a localized complication in the mucosa of the intestine and, only later, leaves some traces on the blood type parameters. However, even in the most important cases, the involvement of allergy-specific antibodies (IgE) is missing and there is no risk of anaphylaxis.

More than a disease, gluten intolerance is preferably defined as a Para physiological condition, since, in the absence of exposure to the specific agent (gluten), the organism remains quietly in homeostasis as if it were healthy. Otherwise, a pathological picture of extremely variable severity and symptoms may arise.

Difference between celiac disease and gluten intolerance

Those who suffer from celiac disease have a very specific type of injury to the intestine, in which the complex proteins of wheat, rye and barley induce the immune system to attack the small intestine, while those who suffer from gluten sensitivity does not have this type of injury, but still feel the inflammation caused by gluten.

The difference between the two disorders is therefore given by the different immune reaction to gluten. In gluten sensitivity, the body's main immune defense (innate immunity) reacts to the ingestion of gluten by fighting it directly, i.e. causing inflammation in the digestive system and other parts of the body. In celiac disease gluten is, instead, fought by both innate and adaptive immunity, that is, by the most sophisticated part of the immune system. Communication problems between the cells of the adaptive immune system cause these cells to fight the tissues of the body, resulting in the atrophy of the intestinal villi associated with celiac disease.

What to eat in case of gluten intolerance

Unfortunately there is no cure for gluten intolerance, but it is possible to live with this condition by following a specific diet, avoiding to consume foods containing this substance. Gluten is found in: wheat, spelt, barley, rye, oats and in all products derived from them such as: bread, pasta, crackers, breadsticks, cookies, cakes, breadcrumbs, yeast, barley coffee and substitutes, malt, beer, soy sauce, cutlets, broth preparations, frying preparations, ice cream preparations and in some cold cuts.

Here is a list of foods that can be consumed by individuals with gluten intolerance:

amaranth, buckwheat, legumes (beans, lentils, peas), corn, millet, quinoa, rice/wheat rice, sesame, soybeans, tapioca, potatoes, chestnuts, all meats, all fish and shellfish, ham, aged cheeses, eggs, vegetables, fruit, butter, lard, extra virgin olive oil, olive oil, peanut oil, soybean oil, corn oil, sunflower oil, grape seed oil, walnut oil, salt and herbs, dried and fresh mushrooms, olives, milk (not mixed with other ingredients), fresh cream, low-fat whole or fruit yoghurt without added cereals or malt, brewer's yeast, roasted ground coffee, tea, chamomile, carbonated soft drinks, nectar and fruit juices, wine, sparkling wine, champagne, grappa, tequila, cognac, brandy, Scotch whisky, cherry, Jamaican rum, port, marsala, sugar, honey.

To be avoided are: Wheat (wheat), spelt, bulgur, oats, kamut, barley, spelt, rye, triticale, sorghum, cous cous, malt and cereal flakes where malt has been added, floured and breaded foods, frozen products (except whole uncleaned fish) if contaminated in processing, surimi, floured nuts, coffee substitutes containing barley, balsamic vinegar, apple cider vinegar, beer, non-Scottish whiskey, vodka, gin and spirits such as bitters, infusions, curry, seitan, cereal and malt yogurt, and soy sauce. For a complete and official list of gluten-free foods suitable for celiac and intolerant people we recommend consulting the AIC handbook: a publication published annually that collects, after evaluation, even products that, although not designed specifically for a particular diet, are still suitable for consumption by celiac.

Desserts

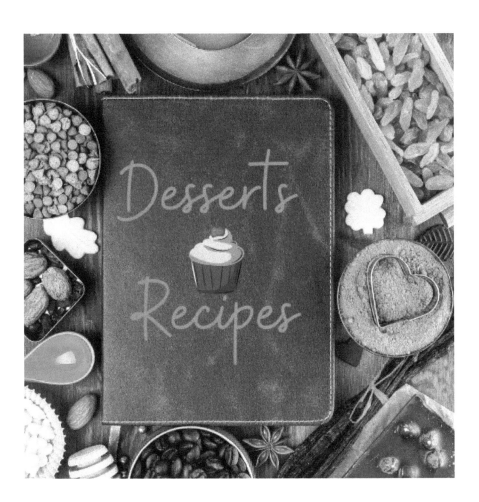

Salted Caramel

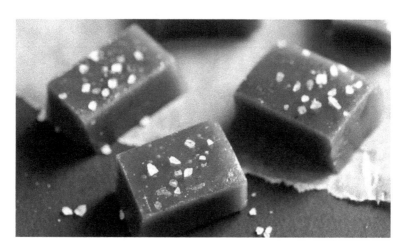

Ingredients for 4 people:

- 100 grams of sugar
- 3 spoons of water
- 250 milliliters of cream
- 40 grams of butter
- fleur de sel de Camargue

Preparation:

1. Start by making the caramel. In a high-sided saucepan, pour the sugar and water. Stir just at the beginning then don't touch the sugar anymore. It will start to become more and more brownish. When it becomes a beautiful bronze color it has reached the optimum temperature.
2. Add the butter a little at a time and stir with a whisk to mix well and bring down the temperature of the caramel a little. Also add the pinch of fior di sale.

3. Now it's time to add the cream. It must be added while continuing to mix with the whisk and dropping it in a trickle, so as to avoid splashes. In a couple of minutes the caramel will have thickened and taken the form of an amber sauce. Pour it into a sterilized preserving jar and let it rest for at least 4 hours. After the resting time it will have changed consistency and will have reached the final more compact and spreadable consistency.

Dried figs stuffed with chocolate

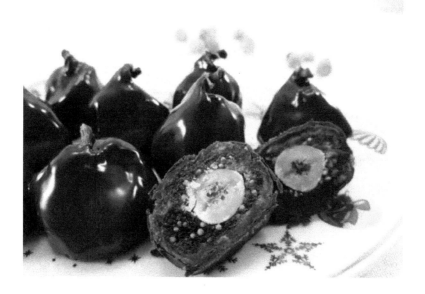

Ingredients for 4 people

- 12 dried figs
- 12 walnut kernels
- 100 grams of dark chocolate to cover

Preparation

1. Prepare all the ingredients and start with the dried figs. With the help of a serrated knife, cut the figs vertically starting from the bottom, and cut them more or less to half their length. With the help of your fingers, soften the figs so that they become malleable and can be stuffed more easily. Now place a walnut kernel inside each fig.
2. Close the figs, taking great care to make the two halves adhere well, so that the cut is not very visible. In a deep

saucepan, pour the dark chocolate for coating, the best for these operations, because it melts quickly, is particularly workable and solidifies very well. Melt the chocolate in a bain-marie, keeping the boiling water at a minimum, until it is completely liquefied.

3. Dip the dried figs stuffed with walnuts in the chocolate, covering only half of it, that is the half that was previously cut, lay them on a sheet of baking paper and let the chocolate cool down becoming solid again. Once they are ready, place them in paper ramekins or in single-portion candy bags.

Caramelized onions

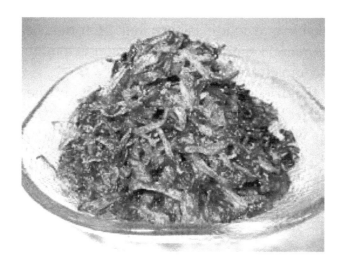

Ingredients for 6 people

- 500 grams of Tropea red onions
- 2 tablespoons of brown sugar
- 1 bay leaf
- 1 pinch of salt
- water
- 50 milliliters of white wine vinegar

Preparation

1. Clean the red onions well of the tougher outer leaves, then slice them into rounds no more than 4 mm thick and place them in a deep bowl. Cover the onions with plenty of cold water and half of the white wine vinegar and let them rest for 60 minutes.
2. After 60 minutes have passed, drain the onions well from the liquid in which they were immersed and rinse them in

clean, cold water, then place them in a pot and continue by adding the brown sugar and bay leaf.

3. Continue adding a pinch of salt to the onions and then add 300 millilitres of water and the leftover wine vinegar, then cover with a lid, turn on the heat and cook for about 45 minutes, stirring from time to time and being careful not to let the cooking liquid dry out too much.

Cream cooked with chocolate

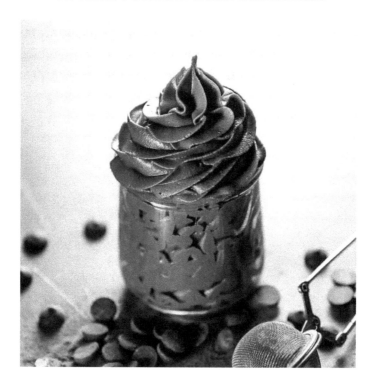

Ingredients for 6 people

- 500 milliliters of fresh liquid cream
- 60 grams of chocolate
- 8 grams of fish glue
- 3 tablespoons of Sugar

Preparation

1. To prepare the panna cotta with chocolate you must take the sheets of isinglass, then fill a jug with 50 millilitres of cold water, dip them in and let them rest 10 minutes.

2. Then take a small saucepan, put the sugar in it and then the cream. Turn on a low flame and bring to a boil. When the cream begins to boil, turn off the heat, squeeze out the isinglass and put it in the saucepan. Stir until it is completely dissolved.

3. Finally, take the Kinder chocolate bars and cut them into rather large flakes. Pour the cream into the molds and add the chocolate.

4. After 5 hours of rest in the refrigerator, the panna cotta with chocolate is ready.

Meringue ghosts

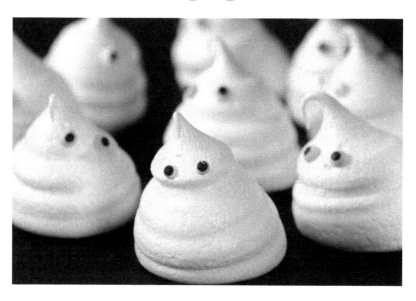

Ingredients for 6 people

- 200 grams of Icing Sugar
- 100 grams of Albumen
- 25 grams of Chocolate

Preparation

1. To prepare the meringue ghosts first you need to split the eggs by separating the whites from the yolks. Then put the egg whites in a planetary mixer and whip them until stiff for a few minutes. Add the powdered sugar one tablespoon at a time while keeping the whisk in action, but moderating the speed.
2. With the help of a ladle fill your sac a poche with the mixture obtained and then form your ghosts in a baking pan covered with parchment paper. Bake at 70 degrees in

a ventilated oven for at least 2 hours. After the time has elapsed, check the cooking by cutting a meringue in half and checking that the center is dry, otherwise put them back in the oven a little more, being careful not to darken the surface.

3. Once cooled, you will have to decorate your ghosts, melt the chocolate and then, with the help of a kitchen pen draw the eyes and mouth.

Cookies with bean flour

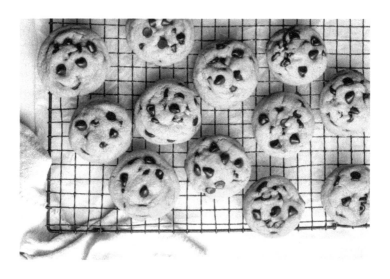

Ingredients for 6 people

- 300 grams of Bean Flour
- 100 grams of Seed Oil
- 50 millilitres of Milk
- 4 tablespoons of Brown Sugar
- 2 Eggs

Preparation

1. To prepare the cookies with bean flour as first thing you have to put the bean flour in a large bowl, then add the seed oil and mix well. Next add the eggs and mix again.
2. Incorporate the brown sugar and whole milk, then form a dough that you will work for a few minutes with your hands.
3. On a pastry board, with the help of a rolling pin, stretch the dough with a thickness of about half a millimetre. Then

with a pastry cup form the cookies and lay them on a baking sheet covered with parchment paper.

4. After 20 minutes of baking at 180 degrees in a static oven here are your cookies with bean flour!

Pineapple Pudding

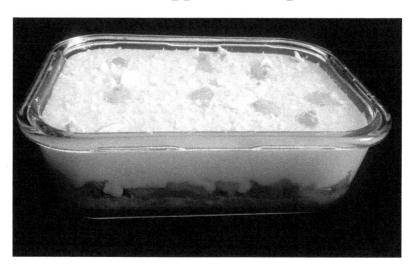

Ingredients for 2 people

- 200 grams of fresh pineapple
- 1 teaspoon of lemon juice
- 1 tablespoon of honey
- 1 yoghurt
- 3 teaspoons of water
- 2 teaspoons of agar agar
- coconut oil

Preparation

1. Cut the pineapple into four similar pieces. Cut the pulp out of one part and put it in a blender. Add a teaspoon of honey and the juice of half a lemon. Blend everything to obtain a frothy and smooth consistency.
2. Pour the water into a small saucepan. Add the agar agar, let it dissolve and then bring to a boil for a moment. Turn

off the heat and add the blended pineapple. Stir everything and let it cool.

3. Finally, add the yogurt. Stir until completely incorporated. Grease a mold with coconut oil and pour the mixture up to the brim. Refrigerate for at least 2 hours.

Mascarpone cream

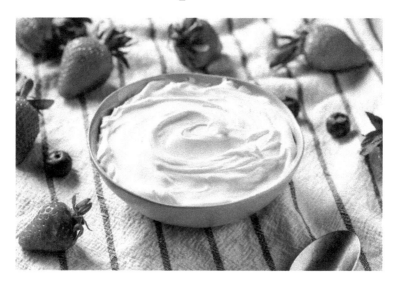

Ingredients for 6 people

- 500 grams of Mascarpone
- 60 grams of sugar
- 20 grams of lukewarm water
- 2 eggs

Preparation

1. To prepare the mascarpone cream as first thing you need to whip the whites to stiff peaks. Break the eggs, put the egg whites in the planetary mixer and beat them until the mixture reaches the consistency of a foam. Then set them aside.
2. Put the egg yolks in the basket, add the sugar and warm water, then mix until the mixture is smooth.

3. Add the mascarpone cheese and work it well until it is completely blended with the eggs and sugar. Then pour it into the bowl where you previously put the whipped whites and gently mix everything together.

4. After two hours of rest in the refrigerator, your mascarpone cream is ready.

Yogurt and blueberry parfait

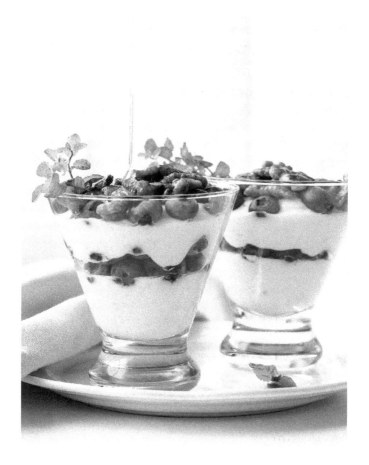

Ingredients for 6 people

- 400 grams of Wild Berries Yogurt
- 150 grams of Cereals
- 30 Blueberries
- 2 tablespoons of Honey
- 1 teaspoon of Brown Sugar
- 1 Lemon

Preparation

1. To prepare the yogurt and blueberry semifreddo, first you need to put the cereals on a cutting board and, with the help of a rolling pin, coarsely reduce them into grains. Then tip them into a bowl and add the honey, mix until everything is well mixed.
2. Take the blueberries, wash them and put them in a bowl, then add the sugar and the juice of half a lemon and mix well.
3. Take a mold and first pour in the blueberries, add the berry yogurt and cover everything with the cereal mixture, arranging them well with your hands.
4. After about 3 hours of rest in the freezer here is your yogurt and blueberry semifreddo.

Chocolates with nuts

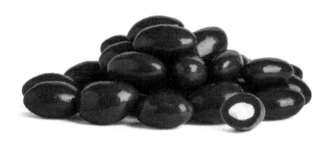

Ingredients for 2 people

- 100 grams of Dark Chocolate
- 80 grams of milk chocolate
- 70 grams of Hazelnuts
- 10 grams of Butter

Preparation

1. This recipe calls for the preparation of 12 nut chocolates. First you need to melt in the microwave or bain-marie the milk chocolate along with the butter.
2. Then put the hazelnuts in the blender, keeping aside 12 for the preparation in step 3, and chop them until they have reached the consistency of a grain. Then pour them into the melted chocolate and mix to amalgamate everything. Place the mixture thus obtained in the refrigerator for 15 minutes.

3. After that time, take everything out of the refrigerator and form small balls with your hands, then place a hazelnut on top of each one.
4. Then melt the dark chocolate and with the help of a grater pour it over each chocolate trying to cover the entire surface.
5. After about 2 hours in the refrigerator to let them cool down.

Coconut Cookies

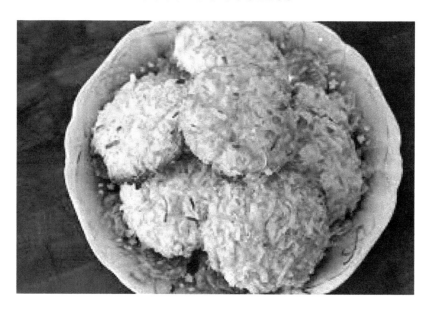

Ingredients for 8 people

- 180 grams of coconut flour
- 100 grams of icing sugar
- 1 sachet of vanillin
- 10 grams of margarine
- 3 egg whites

Preparation

1. In a bowl pour the coconut flour and add the sifted powdered sugar along with the vanillin and mix everything, after which add the melted margarine and resume mixing everything.
2. In a mixer pour the egg whites and whip them until stiff, as soon as they are ready pour the dry ingredients

continuing to work very slowly so that all amalgamates well and being very careful not to disassemble the egg whites. When finished, pour the mixture into a bowl.

3. Wet your palms and, with the help of a teaspoon, portion the mixture into small irregular balls. Place the cookies on a plate and bake at 180 degrees in a static oven for about ten minutes. Once the cookies begin to take color lower the oven to 150 degrees and let them finish baking slowly. As soon as the cookies are cooked, take them out of the oven and remove them from the plate to stop the cooking process. Serve them cold.

Lemon cream without eggs

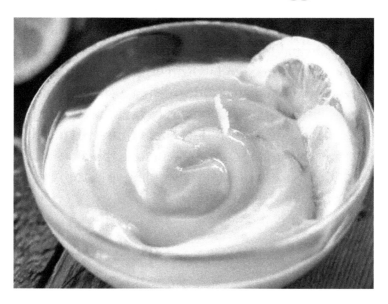

Ingredients for 3 people

- 100 grams of caster sugar
- 20 grams of corn-starch
- 20 grams of rice starch
- 250 grams of fresh milk
- 1 organic lemon
- 30 grams of Butter
- Vanilla seeds

Preparation

1. Pour the caster sugar and the zest of half a lemon into the bimby and chop for 10 seconds at speed 10. Spatulate and repeat the operation in order to obtain a flavoured icing sugar.

2. Add the corn-starch, rice starch, vanilla seeds, fresh milk and cook for 6 minutes at 90 degrees on speed 3.

3. At this point add the butter and cook for another minute at 90 degrees on speed 2. At the end of cooking, add the juice of one filtered lemon and stir for 10 seconds on speed 4.

4. Once cooled, you can serve the lemon cream without eggs with bimby as a spoon dessert or use it for the preparation of cakes and tarts.

Coffee ricotta ice cream

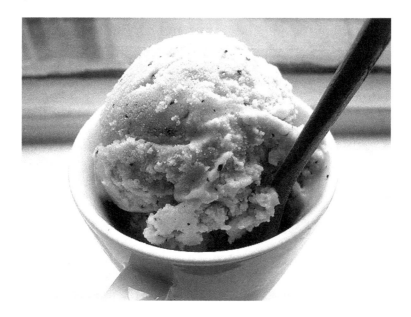

Ingredients for 6 people

- 125 millilitres of water
- 3 spoons of soluble coffee
- 500 grams of ricotta cheese
- 3 eggs
- 100 grams of vanilla sugar
- 4 tablespoons of passito di trani

Preparation

1. Bring the water to a boil and pour the instant coffee into it. Stir to dissolve the powder and allow to cool. Meanwhile, in a large bowl combine the eggs with the vanilla sugar.
2. With an electric mixer, start beating the eggs and sugar until soft and creamy. Add the ricotta and continue

whisking. The ricotta will add extra creaminess to your mixture.

3. Now you need to incorporate the liquid part of the recipe: add the liqueur and the now cold coffee. Pour the mixture into a pitcher so that it can be conveniently poured into the molds. If you opt for a single bowl, pour the cream directly into the container. Put your ice cream in the freezer and let it cool for at least 3 hours. Remember, every hour or so, to stir the mixture in order to break up the ice crystals and obtain a softer cream.

Coconut and chocolate cake without gluten

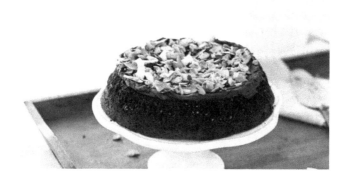

Ingredients for 8 people

-   400 grams of fresh cream
-   250 grams of grated coconut
-   130 grams of caster sugar
-   3 spoons of bitter cocoa
-   3 whole eggs
-   3 teaspoons of baking powder
-   1 sachet of Vanillin

Preparation

1. First pour the cream into a bowl, add the grated coconut, mix well with a spatula until both ingredients are amalgamated. It's the first thing you have to do because while you proceed with the next process the coconut will have time to absorb the cream and moisten well to the right point.

2. Then you can proceed with whipping the eggs, break them into the basket of the planetary mixer, add the sugar and whip them at high speed for at least 5 minutes, until the mixture is clear and frothy. Add the coconut and mix well again until everything is blended.

3. Incorporate the cocoa, vanillin and baking powder and mix for a few more minutes. Pour everything into a baking pan and bake at 180 degrees in a static oven for 25-30 minutes.

4. When you take it out of the oven it will seem rather mushy, but let it cool a bit and your gluten-free coconut and chocolate cake will reach the right consistency and will be ready to be enjoyed.

Cooked cream with coconut milk and lemon

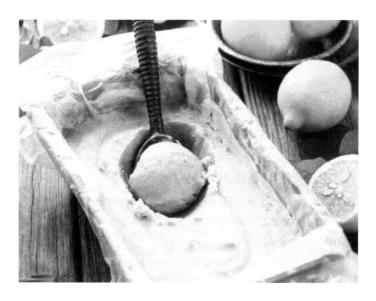

Ingredients for 6 people

- 4 eggs
- 250 millilitres of coconut milk
- 1 tablespoon of lemon essence
- 80 grams of sugar
- strawberries to decorate

Preparation

1. Start by preparing all the ingredients so they are at room temperature. In a bowl, break the eggs and add the sugar.
2. With an electric whisk mix the eggs and sugar until you have a swollen and frothy mixture. Now add the lemon essence. Meanwhile, turn on the oven to 150 degrees and bring it to temperature.

3. Incorporate the coconut milk and stir for another minute to combine all the ingredients well. Pour the mixture into a pitcher so it will be easier to pour the liquid gradually into the molds.

4. Place the muffin or pudding mold in a baking dish. Fill the molds almost to the brim and, in the dish, add 3/4 cup water. Bake them for 40 minutes, then let them cool to room temperature before storing them in the refrigerator for at least 2 hours. Dice the fruit that will accompany your cooked creams.

Apple Teeth

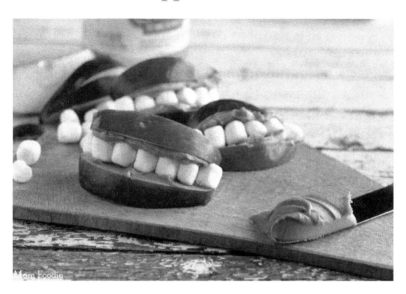

Ingredients for 2 people

- 1 Apple
- 1 tablespoon of Lemon Juice
- 5 Almonds

Preparation

1. Cut almonds into various shapes, creating teeth. Wash and cut the apple in half and then into wedges.
2. Cut off the end without removing the core, which will act as a support. Cut the apple in the middle with two cuts.
3. Remove the inside of the apple. Sprinkle the apple with lemon juice and spread the juice well over the flesh. Pierce the apple to place the almond teeth.

Grilled peaches with cinnamon and rum

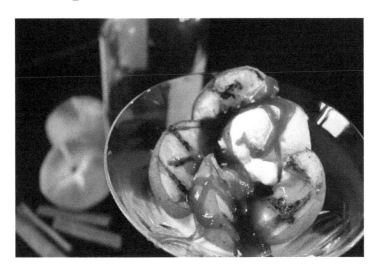

Ingredients for 1 people

- 2 Peaches
- 1 tablespoon of Rum
- 1 tablespoon of Honey
- Cinnamon

Preparation

1. In a bowl, combine the rum and honey. Stir until honey is completely dissolved. Wash and cut the peaches in half.
2. Cut the peaches into slices not too thin, brush them with the rum and honey mixture on both sides and grill two minutes on each side.
3. Turn the slices over, taking care not to burn them, and brush them again with the liquid to make them more succulent. Arrange the slices on a plate and sprinkle with cinnamon. Serve hot.

Cocoa candies with sesame seeds

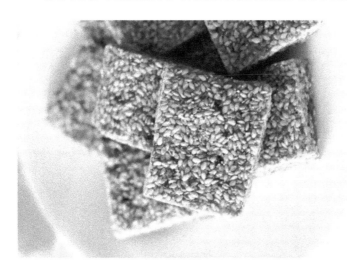

Ingredients for 6 people

- 100 grams of Brown Sugar
- 30 grams of Butter
- 2 teaspoons of sesame seeds
- 1 teaspoon of Bitter Cocoa
- 1 teaspoon of Extra Virgin Olive Oil
- Water

Preparation

1. Pour the sugar into the saucepan and heat over low heat. Add the butter and stir well. Immediately add the sesame seeds, stirring constantly.
2. Add the cocoa and stir to combine well with the caramel. When the mixture thickens, add water and stir until the sugar is completely dissolved.

3. Grease the silicone mold with oil. Pour the caramel into the mold.

4. Tap the mold against the work surface to remove air. Refrigerate for two hours, then remove the caramels from the mold and wrap in plastic wrap.

Figs and hot pepper jam

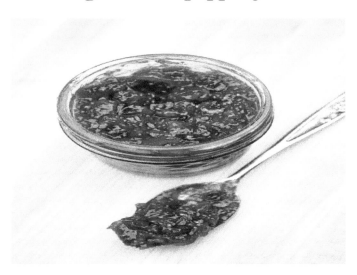

Ingredients for 10 people

- 700 grams of Figs
- 125 grams of sugar
- 30 millilitres of balsamic vinegar
- Chilli pepper

Preparation

1. Start by cleaning the figs, cutting them off at the ends and removing the skin. Cut them into small pieces and place them in a saucepan.
2. Weigh the sugar, pour the balsamic vinegar into a coffee cup and turn on the flame under the fruit. Add the sugar and start swirling to blend the ingredients.
3. Let the fruit cook for 5 minutes, then add the balsamic vinegar and coarsely chopped chili by hand.

4. Cook for another 20 minutes, then blend everything with an immersion blender until all the lumps have disappeared.

Banana split light

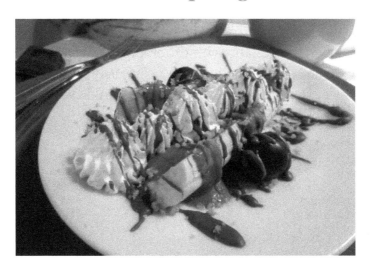

Ingredients for 2 people

- 1 Banana
- 50 grams of Milk Chocolate
- 20 grams of Hazelnuts
- as much as needed of Grapes
- 50 millilitres of Cream
- 60 millilitres of White Yogurt
- 1 teaspoon of Honey
- 2 teaspoons of Bitter Cocoa

Preparation

1. Pour the yogurt into a bowl, add the honey and cocoa. Stir to get a smooth consistency and place in the freezer.
2. Finely chop the hazelnuts. Whip the cream, fill a piping bag and place in the refrigerator.

49

3. Peel the banana and cut it in half, then cut each half lengthwise. Arrange the banana on plates and pour the cooled yogurt between the two banana halves.
4. Garnish the banana with the cream. Using a fork, decorate the cake with the chocolate previously melted in a bain-marie. Decorate with grapes and sprinkle with hazelnuts.

Fig jam

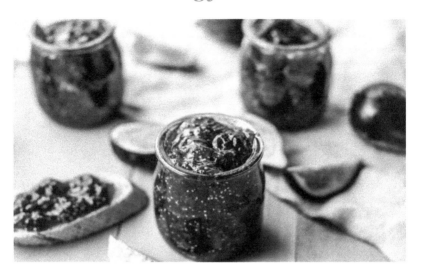

Ingredients for 8 people

- 1 kilo of Figs
- 500 grams of caster sugar
- 20 milliliters of lemon juice

Preparation

1. Wash the figs well and remove the outer skin, weigh them and cut each fruit into at least 4 pieces.
2. Transfer the figs to a saucepan, cover with sugar and stir until combined, then add the lemon juice.
3. Put the fruit on the stove and when it comes to a boil, skim it. Let it cook over low heat for about 45 minutes, taking care not to let it stick. After the time has elapsed, check the cooking by pouring a teaspoon of jam onto a cold plate; if it thickens quickly and remains firm, it will be ready.

4. Pour the jam into jars, turn the jars upside down and leave to cool, then store in a cool place and use within 6 months.

Mango jelly

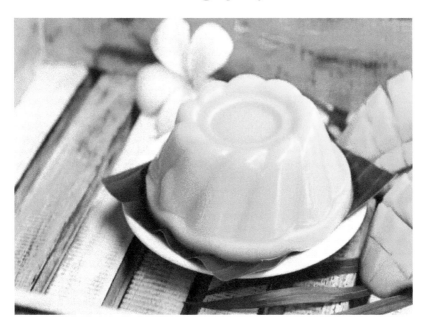

Ingredients for 4 people

- 2 Mango
- 100 millilitres of water
- 7 grams of fish glue

Preparation

1. Wash and peel the mango. Cut it into small pieces and pour over boiling water.
2. Mash the mango with a fork by dipping it well into the water. When it cools down a bit, blend the mixture until it is pureed.
3. Add the isinglass and dissolve it well, stirring until it dissolves completely. Then pour the mixture into a clean

bowl and refrigerate overnight. After the necessary time, cut the gelatine with a sharp knife and use according to preference, i.e. as a dessert or as an ingredient in other sweet recipes.

Blackberry jam

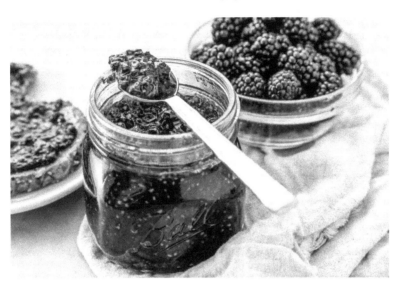

Ingredients for 8 people

- 1 kilo of blackberries
- 600 grams of caster sugar
- 20 milliliters of lemon juice

Preparation

1. Wash the blackberries and let them dry in a colander, then take a third of them and with the help of a blender reduce them to a puree. In a saucepan, add the sugar and the blackberry puree.
2. Add to the sugar and to the puree the whole blackberries and the lemon juice, put the pot on the fire and start cooking the jam for about 30 minutes. As the cooking proceeds, check the density of the jam by transferring a small amount to a cold saucer and letting it slide.

3. Once the jam is ready, transfer it to sterilized jars while still hot, close them and turn them upside down, leaving them like this until they are cold. At this point the jam will be under vacuum until you open your jars to consume it.

Peach jam

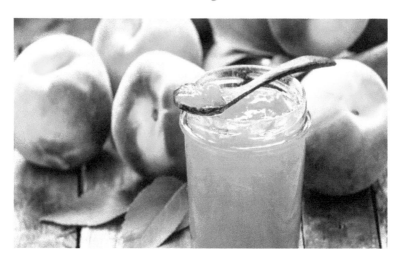

Ingredients for 8 people

- 2 kilos of Peaches
- 1.5 kilos of Sugar
- 1 Lemon

Preparation

1. Peel the peaches and remove the stone, then cut them into small pieces, all more or less the same size, then pour them into a pot and add the sugar and lemon juice. Mix everything together and leave to macerate for at least an hour.
2. After the maceration time has elapsed, turn on the heat to high and bring the peaches to a boil. When the foam forms, foam them well, lower the heat and proceed with the cooking, stirring from time to time, for a time that will vary depending on the wateriness of the fruit from 60 to 90 minutes. In order to be sure of the cooking, do the "saucer

test", that is take a little bit of jam from the pot and let it slide on a cold plate: in this way you will be able to see the degree of wateriness and density and decide whether to continue cooking or not.

3. Once the jam is ready, pot it while it is still hot, in sterile jars, close them and turn them upside down, in this way a vacuum will be created which will serve to make the preserve last longer. Once cold, store them in a cold place and away from light.

Baked peaches with ricotta cream and hazelnuts

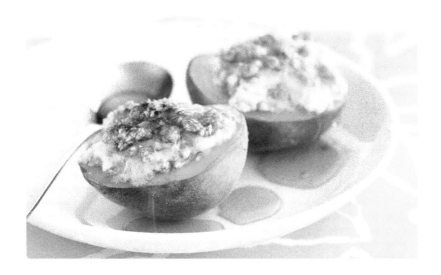

Ingredients for 4 people

- 2 Peaches
- 200 grams of Ricotta
- 10 grams of Sugar
- 80 grams of Chopped Hazelnuts
- 15 milliliters of Maple Syrup
- Cinnamon

Preparation

1. Wash the peaches under running water and cut them in half, removing the stone. Lay them on a baking sheet, skin side up, and cut them with a knife, then transfer them to a preheated oven at 200°C for at least 10 minutes. After the cooking time, turn the peaches upside down from the part

where you removed the stone and make some holes with a toothpick.

2. Sprinkle the peaches with the sugar and then the cinnamon, then put them back in the oven, under the grill, for another 10 minutes. Finally, take them out of the oven and let them cool down.

3. Prepare the ricotta cream by combining it with maple syrup and chopped hazelnuts, mix well and keep it in the fridge so that it cools down before serving the dessert. Compose the dish with the cream and the fruit and sprinkle both with hazelnut crumbs.

Sweet Prickly Pear Salad

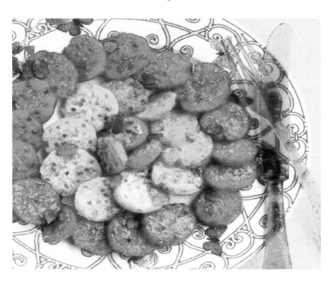

Ingredients for 4 people

- 8 Prickly Pears
- 40 grams of caster sugar
- 30 millilitres of lemon juice
- Mint
- Cinnamon

Preparation

1. In a bowl, pour the sugar, lemon juice and a teaspoon of cinnamon. Stir everything together and let it sit so that the sugar dissolves well.
2. Clean the prickly pears by first placing them in the sink and using rubber gloves, wash them under cold water to remove any thorns. Hold the prickly pear with a hand covered by the glove and with the help of a knife cut the ends, then cut vertically the rest of the skin and with the hand without the glove gently extract the fruit.

3. Place the cleaned fruit on a cutting board, cut slices at least 4 mm thick and place them in a bowl.
4. Season the prickly pears with the chopped mint and the sugar and lemon dressing prepared earlier. Mix everything together and let stand in the fridge for half an hour, then serve.

Mini pavlova with ice cream

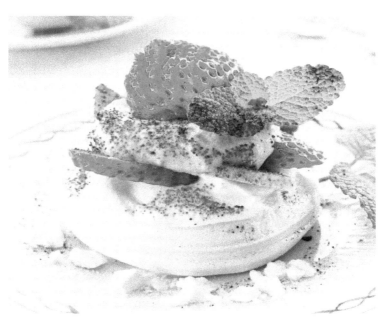

Ingredients for 6 people

- 60 grams of egg whites
- 60 grams of Icing Sugar
- 60 grams of caster sugar
- 6 tablespoons of ice cream

Preparation

1. Preheat the oven to 110 °C. Separate the yolks from the egg whites and weigh the latter. Weigh the same amount of powdered sugar and granulated sugar.
2. Combine the two sugars in the same bowl and mix them lightly together. Whip the egg whites until stiff. Preparation will take just over 5 minutes.
3. In a bowl combine the whites with the sugars, adding a little at a time and mixing them from the bottom up not to

deflate the mixture. You should obtain a shiny and homogeneous mixture.

4. Line a baking sheet with greaseproof paper and, with the help of a spoon, place small mounds of the mixture quite far apart. Lower the center of the meringue with the wet spoon and bake for about 60 minutes. The heat of the oven should dry out the meringues. They will be ready when they begin to crack slightly on the surface. Remove from oven and allow to cool. Serve with a scoop of black cherry variegated ice cream.

Mango Chutney

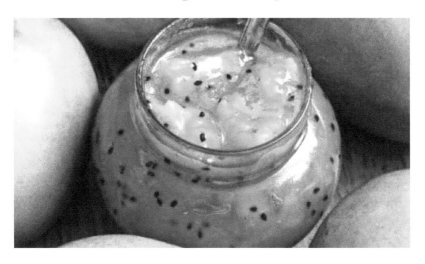

Ingredients for 2 people

- 1 Mango
- 1 Red Onion
- 2 Cloves of Garlic
- 1 glass of Brown Sugar
- 1 glass of Apple Vinegar
- 30 grams of Ginger
- 12 Cardamom seeds
- 1 teaspoon of Turmeric
- 1 pinch of hot chili powder
- 1 pinch of Cinnamon
- 1 teaspoon of Cumin
- 1 teaspoon of Coriander
- 1 tablespoon Extra Virgin Olive Oil

Preparation

1. Wash, peel and dice the mango.

2. Wash, peel and cut the onion into vertical slices. Cut the garlic and put it together with the onion in a pan, then add the oil and sugar. Fry for a couple of minutes, stirring constantly.
3. Add the vinegar and turn up the heat. Wash, peel and finely chop the ginger. Peel the cardamom seeds. Add to the mixture in the pot and bring to a boil.
4. Lower the heat and add the turmeric, chili and cinnamon.
5. Also add the cumin and coriander seeds. Stir well and finally add the mango. Combine well with the spicy mixture. Cover with a lid and cook about 60-70 minutes on low heat, stirring occasionally. Cool and place in a glass jar. Store in the refrigerator and serve cold as an accompaniment to different dishes.

Eton mess

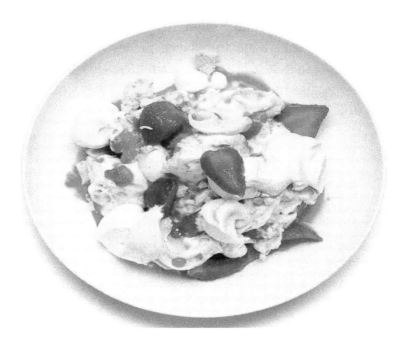

Ingredients for 4 people

- 150 grams of Meringue
- 150 grams of Strawberries
- 250 grams of Fresh Cream
- 70 grams of Icing Sugar
- 1 teaspoon of Vanilla extract

Preparation

1. Wash the strawberries in water lightly acidulated, with lemon or vinegar, and dry them well. Clean them and cut them into pieces. Transfer half of the strawberries to a bowl and mash them with a fork.

2. Whip the cream with the sugar and vanilla, then roughly incorporate the crushed strawberries, making sure not to put the juice they have released.
3. Break the meringue into large pieces and assemble the cake by placing a layer of meringues, one of cream and strawberries in pieces. Continue in this way until the glass is full.

Strawberry soufflé

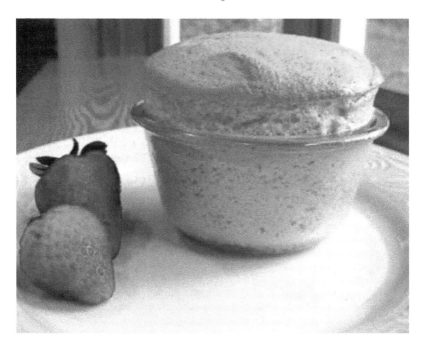

Ingredients for 2 people

- 130 grams of Strawberries
- 60 grams of Brown Sugar
- 2 Albumens
- 1 teaspoon of seed oil
- 1 Lemon

Preparation

1. Grease two soufflé molds with oil. Wash the strawberries and put them in a blender. Add the juice of half a lemon and blend to obtain a smooth and homogeneous mixture.

2. In a tall saucepan, previously chilled in the fridge, pour the egg whites. Add the sugar and beat the egg whites until stiff.

3. Add the strawberry smoothie and stir gently from top to bottom so as not to disassemble the egg whites. Fill the moulds up to 3/4 of their capacity and bake in a preheated oven at 200 °C, then lower the temperature to 190 °C and bake for a maximum of 10 minutes. The soufflés should puff up as they go over the edge. Once baked, they will sink a little. They can be served high and hot or cold with fresh strawberries.

Apricot tart gluten free

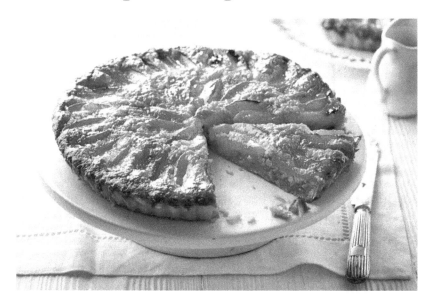

Ingredients for 6 people

- 250 grams of rice flour
- 150 grams of corn flour
- 2 Eggs
- 180 grams of Brown Sugar
- 150 grams of Butter
- Water
- 1 pinch of Salt
- 7 Apricots

Preparation

1. On a work surface, pour the two flours, cold butter in small pieces, room temperature eggs and sugar. Mix with a silicone spatula or fork and then work a little with your

hands. Form a ball, wrap it in plastic wrap and refrigerate for half an hour.

2. Take the shortbread out of the fridge. Leave aside a small piece of dough, put the remaining part on a work surface sprinkled with cornmeal and roll out a sheet not too fine with the help of a rolling pin. Transfer the pastry sheet to the buttered baking pan and sprinkle with sugar.

3. Prick with a fork, wash and cut in half the apricots and place them on the pastry, trying to cover the entire surface.

4. Sprinkle the apricots with brown sugar. Roll out the leftover dough and cut strips of about 1,5 - 2 cm. Place the strips on top of the fruit and brush with sugar water. Bake in a preheated oven at 180 °C for about 25-30 minutes. Let cool and serve.

Mascarpone cream with coffee and brandy

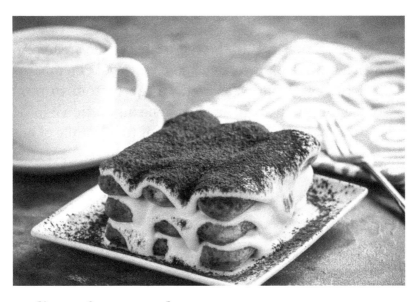

Ingredients for 4 people

- 250 grams of Mascarpone
- 4 eggs
- 100 grams of Sugar
- 1 tablespoon of Soluble Coffee
- 2 spoons of Brandy

Preparation

1. Separate the yolk and white of the egg. In a tall bowl, whisk the egg whites until stiff. Start on speed one and beat like this for a good minute, then move to speed two for another minute. Check to make sure your egg whites are well whipped.
2. In another bowl, add the sugar and instant coffee to the egg yolks. Start whipping for 5 minutes, until the mixture is frothy and fluffy.

3. Add the two tablespoons of brandy and the mascarpone to the cream. Whip again to mix the liquid well into your mixture.

4. The last step is to add the egg whites to the cream. Add it with a spatula or a wooden spoon, always remembering to mix the egg whites gently from the bottom to the top. When the mixture will be homogeneous portion it into four glasses and put it in the refrigerator for a couple of hours.

Banana mousse with hot chocolate

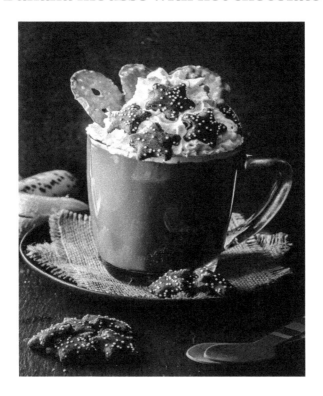

Ingredients for 4 people

- 2 Bananas
- 250 milliliters of fresh cream
- 3 teaspoons of cane sugar
- Lemon Juice
- 50 grams of dark chocolate

Preparation

1. Pour the cream into a large bowl, previously cooled. Whip it until stiff, but not too hard, with the help of electric whips, then place it in the fridge.

2. Pour the sugar into the saucepan. Cut the bananas into slices, not too thick, and add them to the sugar. Caramelise them over low heat until the sugar has dissolved, stirring constantly. Refrigerate for 5 minutes.

3. When the bananas have cooled, blend them to a creamy, smooth consistency. Add a squeeze of lemon. Finally, add the cream and whisk with electric whips at a medium speed to blend the ingredients well, but do not disassemble the cream.

4. Melt the chocolate in a bain-marie. Place the mousse in a piping bag and fill the cups. Pour over the hot chocolate and serve immediately.

Sicilian lemon granita

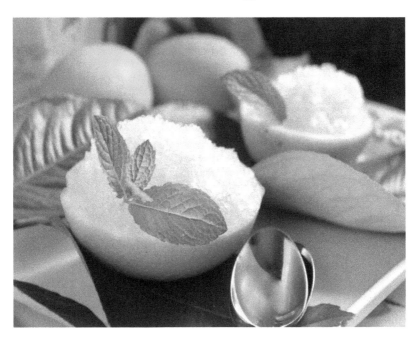

Ingredients for 4 people

- 200 millilitres of lemon juice
- 500 millilitres of water
- 300 grams of caster sugar

Preparation

1. Place a small saucepan on the stove and melt the sugar with the water until you have a liquid syrup.
2. Strain the lemon juice and pour it into the saucepan with the lukewarm syrup, then stir everything and place it in the refrigerator for at least 6 hours or until it becomes very cold.

3. Once the liquid has cooled, prepare your ice cream maker for use, then refrigerate the basket and insert the liquid inside. Start the machine and let the syrup thicken forming the granita, which will be ready in about 50 minutes, then serve it in iced cups.

French style meringues

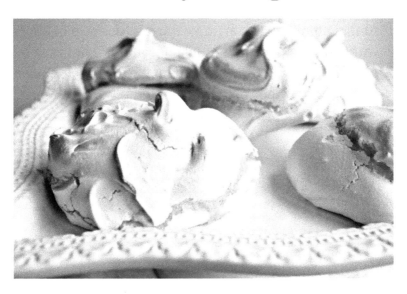

Ingredients for 4 people

- 100 grams of egg whites
- 150 grams of Icing Sugar
- 1 teaspoon of lemon juicee

Preparation

1. Turn on the oven to 90 °C in fan mode. Sift the icing sugar. Start whipping the egg whites with the lemon juice, doubling their volume by at least 3 times.
2. At that point you can start adding a little bit of powdered sugar, always continuing to whisk, when it will be all incorporated continue to whisk for at least 10 minutes. When you get a very smooth, shiny and dense dough you can stop whipping and check the consistency by dipping

the whisk off: withdrawing it on the compound should remain attached forming the classic goose beak.

3. At this point you can arrange the mixture on a baking sheet with the help of a spoon. Bake for about 2 hours at 90 ° C, after the cooking time leave them in the oven for at least 12 hours, so that they will dry completely.

Rice milk sorbet with peaches and coconut

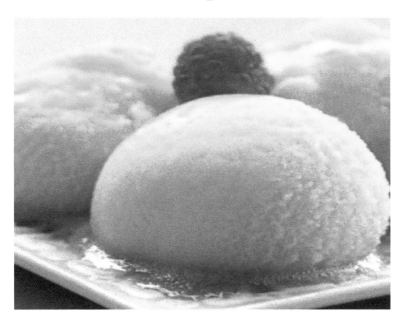

Ingredients for 4 people

- 500 millilitres of rice milk
- 30 grams of Coconut
- 1 Peach
- 1 tablespoon of Honey

Preparation

1. Wash and puncture the coconut. Let out all the water and break the shell with a dish towel. Extract the pulp, remove the brown skin and chop it finely.
2. Pour the rice milk into a blender. Add the coconut and honey. Blend to obtain a homogeneous mixture. Pour it into a baking dish and transfer it to the freezer for 2 hours.

3. Wash the peach. Cut one half into thin slices, which you will use to garnish your sorbet. The other half peel it and cut it into small cubes.
4. Take the pan out of the freezer. Using a spoon, scrape the surface of the sorbet. Put the peach and the sorbet in the blender and blend for a few seconds to combine the ingredients and break up the ice balls. Serve immediately with the peach slices.

Homemade almond milk

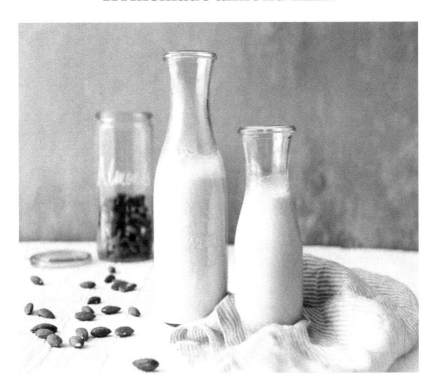

Ingredients for 2 people

- 300 grams of Almonds
- 1 liter of Water

Preparation

1. Blanch the almonds in boiling water and remove the brown film covering them.
2. Blend the almonds with a little water until smooth and fairly smooth.
3. Pour the mixture into a glass bowl, add the hot water and let stand for 2 hours.

83

4. Strain the mixture through a sieve (even 2 times if you have patience) or a clean cloth and pour the milk obtained in a glass bottle.

Creme caramel

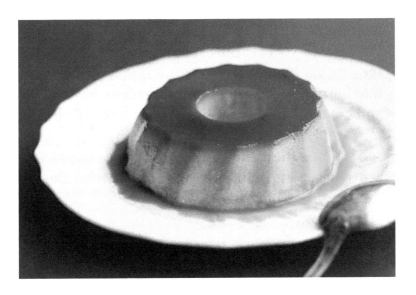

Ingredients for 4 people

- 4 Eggs
- 2 Yolks
- 160 grams of Sugar
- 650 millilitres of Milk
- 1 teaspoon of Vanilla extract
- 100 grams of Sugar for the caramel
- Oil

Preparation

1. Heat the milk, but do not bring it to a boil. Add the sugar and vanilla to the eggs and mix well with a wooden spoon.
2. Add the hot milk to the egg and sugar mixture and stir well so that all the sugar is dissolved. Lightly oil the molds.

3. Prepare the caramel by putting a layer of sugar in a pan, let it caramelize, stir slightly and add more sugar. Continue in this way until all the sugar has been used up.

4. Put a light layer of caramel at the base of each mold. Strain the egg, milk and sugar mixture into a pitcher and pour into the molds. Place the molds in a high-sided baking dish and tap them to remove air bubbles. Bake in a bain-marie for 30 minutes at 180°C and for another 20 minutes at 160°C. After the creme caramel has cooled completely, you can turn it out onto a plate to serve. With the leftover caramel you could make sugar decorations and place them on the cake.

Baked spiced apple

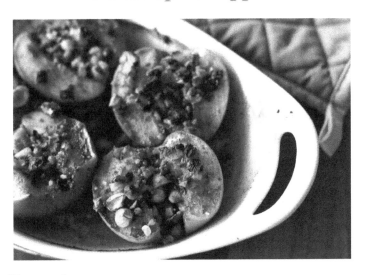

Ingredients for 1 person

- 1 Apple
- 1 teaspoon of Raisins
- 1 teaspoon of Rum
- 1 teaspoon of Cinnamon
- 1 teaspoon of Wild Berry Jam
- 1 Lemon
- 1 Tangerine
- 2 teaspoons of Brown Sugar
- 1 teaspoon of Cloves

Preparation

1. Wash the apple and cut off the top. Remove the apple stem.
2. Also remove some of the flesh and cut it into small pieces. Sprinkle the apple with lemon juice, including the top, and sprinkle with sugar.
3. Prepare the filling: combine the chopped apple with the jam, cinnamon and tangerine juice in a bowl.

4. Add the rum and raisins. Mix well, let macerate 15 minutes and then fill the apple.

5. With a toothpick make holes in the top of the apple and insert the cloves. Sprinkle with sugar, cover the apple and place it on baking paper. Bake at 170 °C for 40 minutes. Serve piping hot.

Hazelnut cream without sugar

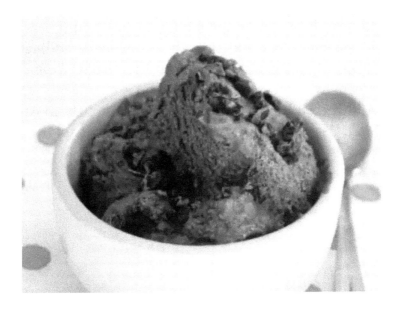

Ingredients for 2 people

- 150 grams of Hazelnuts
- 2 teaspoons of Honey
- 40 millilitres of Coconut Water
- 30 millilitres of Olive Oil
- 20 millilitres of lukewarm water
- 3 grams of Salt
- 2 grams of Bicarbonate

Preparation

1. Shell and clean the hazelnuts and chop them finely. Add the salt and chop for another minute.
2. Add the baking soda and grind another three minutes or so, after which add the honey. Grind another three

minutes, then transfer the hazelnut paste to a bowl and pour over the coconut water. Mix everything together well.

3. Return the cream to the food processor and process until it becomes clear and smooth, occasionally adding a few drops of warm water to soften the cream. Transfer the cream to a bowl.

4. Add the oil to the cream and stir vigorously to combine well. Use coconut water to adjust the density of the cream.

Pear Chutney

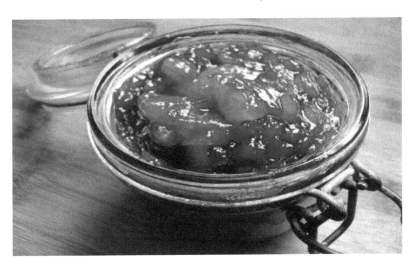

Ingredients for 4 people

- 2 Pears
- 1 Lemon
- 1 teaspoon of Vinegar
- 100 grams of Sugar (half the weight of the fruit)
- Salt
- Mint

Preparation

1. Wash and peel the pears. Cut them and place them in a saucepan.
2. Add the sugar, vinegar and lemon and stir well. Bring the fruit to a boil, then lower the heat and let it cook for at least 20-25 minutes.
3. While cooking you will see that the pears will begin to soften and become shinier, just like in the preparation of

jam. To make the mixture more homogeneous you might stir with a whisk. Once the conserve has thickened slightly it will be ready, then transfer it to a bowl and let it cool completely before serving, with a few leaves of mint to enhance the flavor.

Mint panna cotta with vodka and dark chocolate

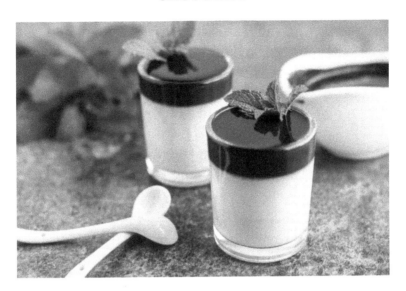

Ingredients for 4 people

- 200 millilitres of cream
- 5 grams of fish glue
- 40 millilitres of milk
- 40 grams of Brown Sugar
- 15 millilitres of Vodka
- 10 grams of Fresh Mint
- 5 grams of Dark Chocolate

Preparation

1. Soak the isinglass in cold water for 10 minutes. Pull the mint leaves off the sprig and pound them with the help of a mortar.
2. Pour the milk into the saucepan, add the cream and dip half of the mint leaves in it. Heat over medium heat for 5-7 minutes, but do not let the mixture boil.

Cover the other half of the mint leaves with vodka and let it macerate.

3. Pour the milk through a strainer into a large bowl. Pound the leaves to release all the liquid. Add the brown sugar and stir until dissolved. Squeeze the isinglass well and add it to the milk, letting it dissolve well.

4. Aggiungete la vodka, strizzando bene le foglie di menta. Grattugiate il cioccolato fondente, aggiungetelo al composto senza però mescolare e riempite gli stampini leggermente unti di olio, dopodiché cospargete sopra ancora con il cioccolato grattugiato. Mettete in frigo per almeno 6 ore, ma meglio per tutta la notte. Guarnite con la menta fresca e delle scaglie di cioccolato fondente.

Gluten free shortcrust pastry

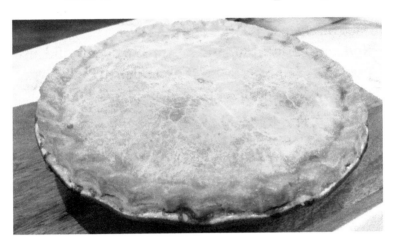

Ingredients for 4 people

- 300 grams of rice flour
- 150 grams of fine corn flour
- 2 Eggs
- 175 grams of Sugar
- 150 grams of Butter
- Milk
- Salt

Preparation

1. Mix well the two types of flour and place them in a fountain on a pastry board. Add the sugar, eggs, soft butter in pieces, a pinch of salt, a little milk and start mixing the ingredients first with the help of a fork and then with your hands.
2. Knead until you get a compact and homogeneous dough, without the need to work it too long. Wrap it in plastic

wrap and let it rest in the refrigerator for about an hour. After this time, take the dough out of the fridge and put it back on the pastry board.

3. Roll out a thin but not too much dough and use it to prepare a delicious tart or classic shortbread cookies, then bake in a preheated oven at 180 ° C for about 20-25 minutes.

English style pears with white chocolate mousse

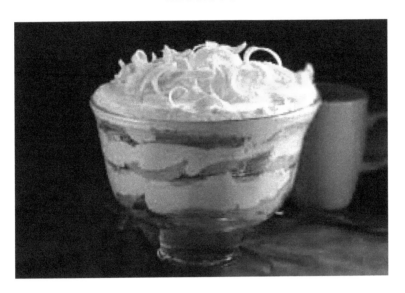

Ingredients for 4 people

- 3 Pears
- 1 litre of water
- 20 grams of Sugar
- 70 grams of Dark Chocolate
- 50 grams of White Chocolate
- 25 millilitres of Milk
- 75 milliliters of Cream

Preparation

1. In a saucepan put the water and sugar and boil for about 10 minutes. Peel and cut the pears in half and remove the core, place them in a bowl and pour the prepared water syrup over them. Leave them like this for a few minutes.

2. Prepare the mousse by melting the white chocolate in a bain-marie, heat the milk until simmering, not boiling, and pour it over the chocolate, stir and leave to one side to cool. Whip the cream.

3. Add the cream to the now cooled chocolate and milk, using a slow but firm motion from top to bottom. Melt the dark chocolate in a bain-marie and let it cool. Drain the pears and dry the excess water with kitchen paper, compose the dish combining the pears with the mousse and the melted dark chocolate, not hot.

Toffee Caramel Sauce

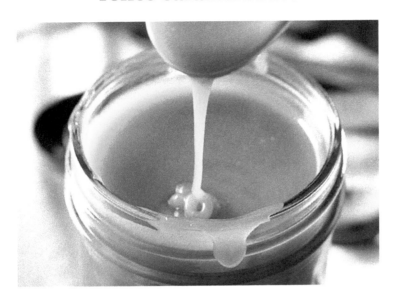

Ingredients for 4 people

- 300 millilitres of cream
- 50 grams of cane sugar
- 30 grams of Butter

Preparation

1. In a small saucepan melt the brown sugar, begin to lower the heat when caramel begins to form.
2. Once all the sugar has become caramel, quickly add the cream which you have heated in another saucepan or in the microwave, being careful not to stand too close to the saucepan as it may give off some very strong steam.
3. Boil for about 8 minutes, until the mixture has thickened and darkened. Once the heat is off, add the butter and stir until melted. Once ready transfer the caramel to a jar, best

sterilized if you want to keep it for a long time, but let it cool a bit before using it as it may be very hot.

Apple and Cinnamon Jam

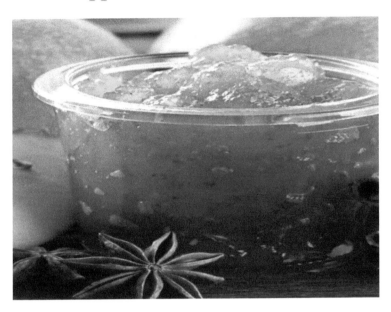

Ingredients for 4 people

- 1 kilo of Apples
- 350 grams of caster sugar
- 1 Lemon
- 2 spoons of Cinnamon

Preparation

1. Wash the apples and cut them into pieces after removing the skin and core. Put them in a blender and run it for a while to obtain very small pieces of apple, not a real smoothie.
2. Transfer to a saucepan along with the sugar and lemon juice, stir and let stand for about 10-15 minutes.

3. In the meantime sterilize some jars whose total capacity should be about one kilo. To do this, boil the jars, lids and possible seals in a pot filled with water up to the height of the jars. Leave the jars in the water until ready to use.

4. Place the saucepan on the stove, bring to a boil and, stirring constantly, cook over low heat for about 40 minutes, or until the mixture has thickened. A few minutes before turning off the heat, add the cinnamon.

5. Transfer the jam into sterilized jars, close them hermetically and turn them upside down to create a vacuum. Alternatively, boil them for about ten minutes in a large pot completely covered with water.

Pumpkin and Ginger Jam

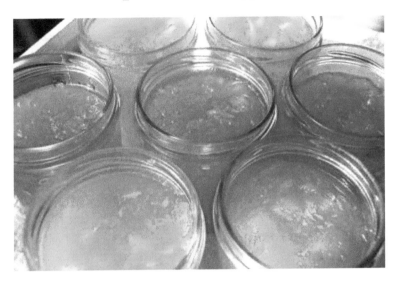

Ingredients for 6 people

- 1 kilo of cleaned pumpkin
- 30 grams of Ginger
- 1 Lemon
- 300 grams of Brown Sugar
- 300 grams of caster sugar

Preparation

1. Clean the pumpkin by removing the outer skin as well as the seeds and the internal filaments. Cut the pumpkin into small pieces, wash it well and place it in a large bowl. Pour into it the brown sugar, the caster sugar and the juice of half a lemon. Mix everything together quickly, cover with plastic wrap and let it rest for at least three hours.

2. In the meantime, sterilize some jars whose total capacity should be about one kilo. To do this, put the jars, lids and any seals in a pot, fill it with water until it exceeds the height of the jars, bring to a boil and leave them immersed in water until ready to use.

3. Take the fresh ginger root, peel it and grate it finely.

4. Once the three hours are up, pour the pumpkin mixture, lemon juice and sugar into a saucepan. Add the grated ginger, stir well and bring the mixture to a boil. Once the mixture comes to a boil, lower the heat and continue cooking, stirring continuously, for about 40 minutes, or until the mixture thickens.

5. Pour the jam into jars, close them well and create a vacuum by turning them upside down or boiling them for ten minutes in a large pot completely covered with water.

Strawberry jam

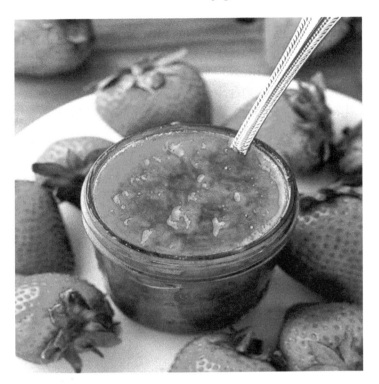

Ingredients for 6 people

- 1 kilo of Strawberries
- 1 Lemon
- 800 grams of Sugar

Preparation

1. Wash the strawberries, remove the stem and cut them into four parts. Place them in a large bowl with the sugar and lemon juice, mix well, cover with plastic wrap and let stand for a couple of hours.

2. In the meantime, sterilize some jars whose total capacity should be about 1.5 kg. To do this, place jars, lids and any seals in a saucepan large enough to fill with water up to the height of the jars. Bring to a boil and leave them submerged in the water until ready to use.

3. After the two hours have passed, pour the mixture into a saucepan, bring to a boil and stir continuously until the jam has reached the right density.

4. Pour the jam into jars, close them well and create a vacuum by turning them upside down or boiling them for ten minutes in a large pot completely covered with water.

Gluten-free cookies with jam

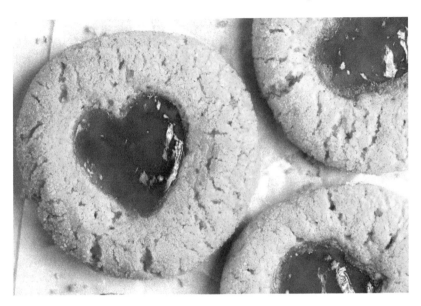

Ingredients for 6 people

- 3 teaspoons of bitter cocoa powder
- 40 grams of hazelnut flour
- 50 grams of buckwheat flour
- 50 grams of fine corn flour
- 50 grams of chestnut flour
- 50 grams of rice flour
- 80 grams of Brown Sugar
- 40 grams of Sunflower Seed Oil
- 1 Egg
- Water
- 1 teaspoon of baking powder
- 1 pinch of Salt
- Jam of your choice

Preparation

1. In a bowl pour all the dry ingredients, so the rice flour, fine corn flour, buckwheat flour, hazelnut flour, chestnut flour, cocoa powder, brown sugar, pinch of salt and baking powder and mix. In the center, add the sunflower oil and mix with your hands, incorporating it into the other ingredients and creating a sandy mixture.

2. Add the beaten egg and knead until you get a dough similar to a shortbread. If it is too dry, add a few tablespoons of water. Since they do not have butter, these cookies do not need to rest so they can be worked right away, but if you prefer an easier to handle mixture you can let it rest in the refrigerator for half an hour. Then lay the cookie mixture on a floured surface.

3. Using a rolling pin, roll out the dough and cut out cookies using cookie cutters suitable for making bull's-eyes. Otherwise make your favorite shapes in pairs and pierce one of the pairs in the center with a smaller shape, even a cup will do. Lay the pierced disc on top of the whole one and fill the center with a teaspoon of jam. Bake the gluten-free cookies in a hot oven at 170 degrees for about 12 minutes.

4. Once cooled, serve your gluten-free cookies with jam for a healthy and original snack or breakfast.

Trifle zucchini

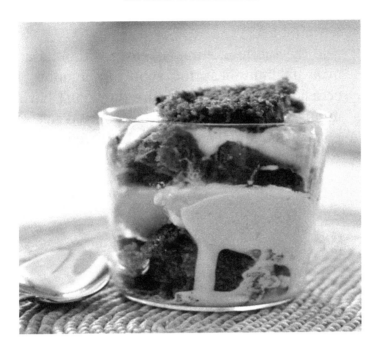

Ingredients for 4 people

- 3 Courgettes
- 1 clove of Garlic
- 1 handful of Parsley
- Extra Virgin Olive Oil
- Salt and Pepper

Preparation

1. Wash the zucchini, cut off the two ends, cut them first in half lengthwise and then into strips about an inch thick. Cut each of these into two to three parts depending on the length of the zucchini.

2. In a pan, preferably non-stick, pour two tablespoons of extra virgin olive oil, add a clove of garlic and fry for a few minutes.

3. Add the zucchini, stir well, cover with a lid and cook over medium heat for about 15 minutes, stirring occasionally and making sure they don't burn. A few minutes before the end of cooking, add salt, chopped parsley and a pinch of pepper. Stir well and serve the zucchini piping hot.

Buttercream

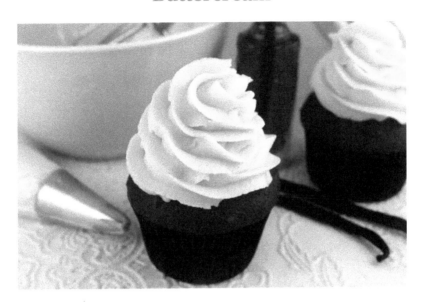

Ingredients for 4 people

- 150 grams of Butter
- 150 grams of Icing Sugar

Preparation

1. Sift the powdered sugar into a bowl. Lightly cream the room temperature butter, then add half of the sugar and mix with a spatula.
2. Whip the mixture with an electric whisk until very light and clear, then add more powdered sugar and continue to whip. To prevent the powdered sugar from getting everywhere, protect the bowl with a clean tea towel. Next, whip the butter with the remaining sugar until the mixture is very smooth and homogeneous.

APPENDIX

Cooking Conversion Charts

Volume (liquid)	
US Customary	Metric
1/8 teaspoon	0,6 ml
1/4 teaspoon	1.2 ml
1/2 teaspoon	2.5 ml
3/4 teaspoon	3.7 ml
1 teaspoon	5 ml
1 tablespoon	15 ml
2 tablespoon or 1 fluid ounce	30 ml
1/4 cup or 2 fluid ounces	59 ml
1/3 cup	79 ml
1/2 cup	118 ml
2/3 cup	158 ml
3/4 cup	177 ml
1 cup or 8 fluid ounces	237 ml
2 cups or 1 pint	473 ml
4 cups or 1 quart	946 ml
8 cups or 1/2 gallon	1.9 litres
1 gallon	3.8 litres

Weight (mass)	
US contemporary (ounces)	Metric (grams)
1/2 ounce	14 grams
1 ounce	28 grams
3 ounces	85 grams
3.53 ounces	100 grams
4 ounces	113 grams
8 ounces	227 grams
12 ounces	340 grams
16 ounces or 1 pound	454 grams

Oven Temperatures	
US contemporary	Metric
250° F	121° C
300° F	149° C
350° F	177° C
400° F	204° C
450° F	232° C

Volume Equivalents (liquid)

3 teaspoons	1 tablespoon	0.5 fluid ounce
2 tablespoons	1/8 cup	1 fluid ounce
4 tablespoons	1/4 cup	2 fluid ounces
5 1/3 tablespoons	1/3 cup	2.7 fluid ounces
8 tablespoons	1/2 cup	4 fluid ounces
12 tablespoons	3/4 cup	6 fluid ounces
16 tablespoons	1 cup	8 fluid ounces
2 cups	1 pint	16 fluid ounces
2 pints	1 quart	32 fluid ounces
4 quarts	1 gallon	128 fluid ounces

CPSIA information can be obtained
at www.ICGtesting.com
Printed in the USA
LVHW021531110521
687091LV00003B/418